VBAC Wizard
Training Manual

School of the Birth Wizardry
Tome of Birth Wisdom
Volume IIII: VBAC Wizard

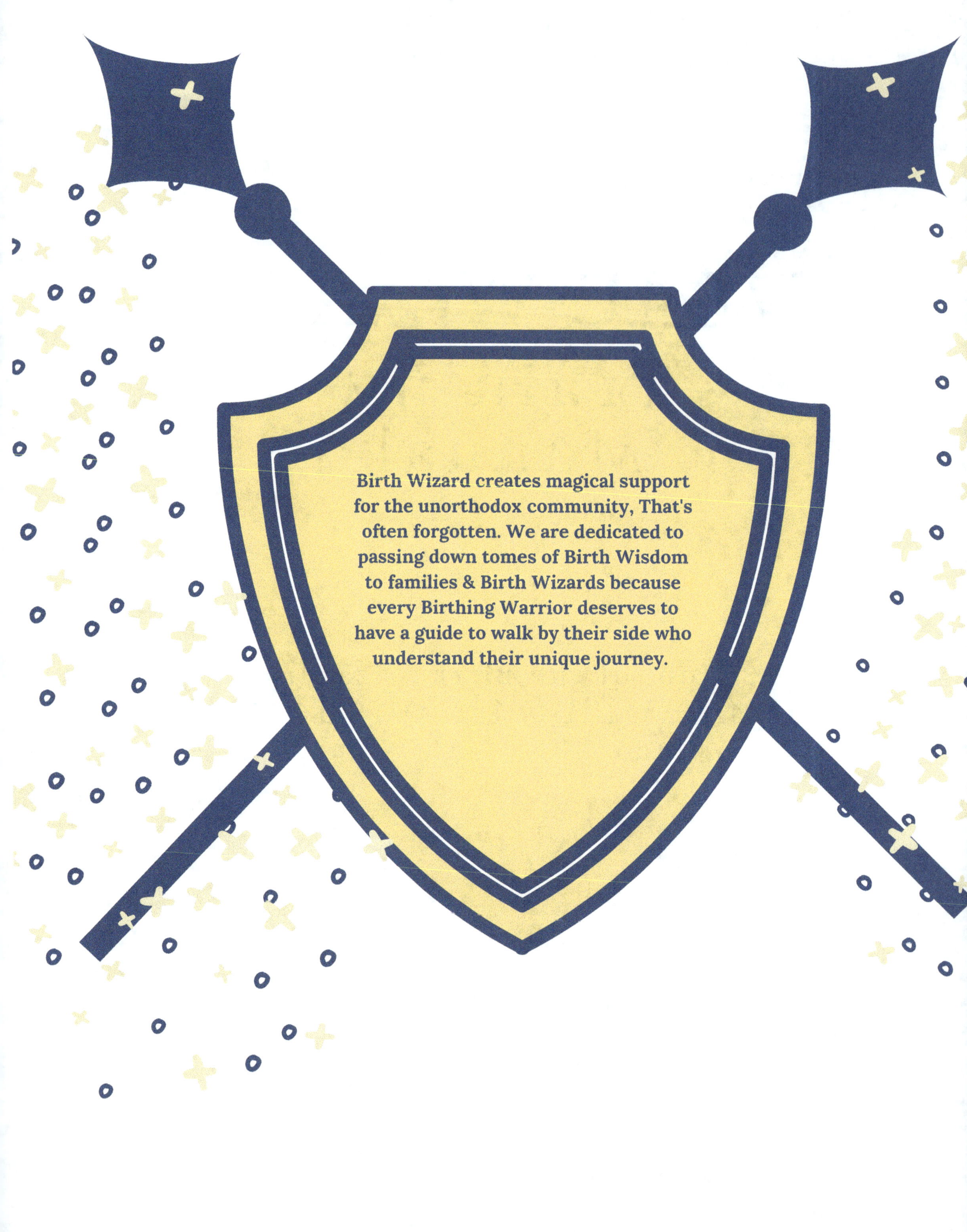

Birth Wizard creates magical support for the unorthodox community, That's often forgotten. We are dedicated to passing down tomes of Birth Wisdom to families & Birth Wizards because every Birthing Warrior deserves to have a guide to walk by their side who understand their unique journey.

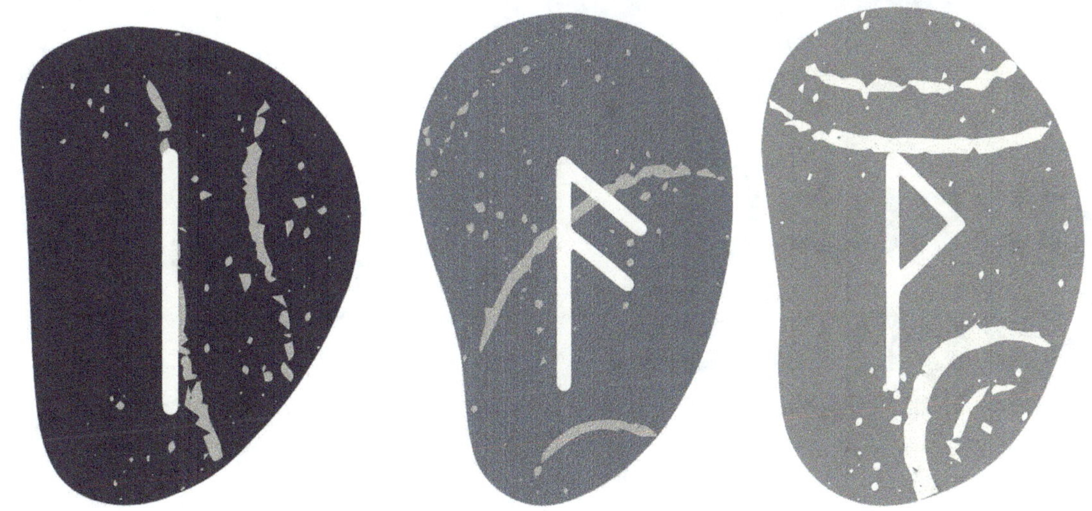

Table of Contents

Huzzah! Welcome!

I appreciate you taking this unique class to enrich your knowledge and helping others through their VBAC journey. This class was developed with care, understanding and knowing how important this is to you. My own quest for VBAC is what led me to be an advocate, doula and educator.

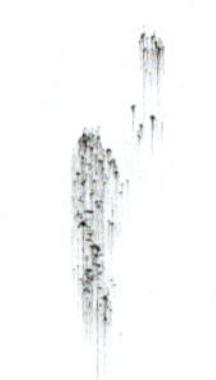

My first pregnancy "was a dream" and I assumed that childbirth would be the same. I was the "perfect patient", meaning never questioned anything the doctor's or hospital told me, and like 1 in 3 women in America, this resulted in a Cesarean. The operative report from Cesarean references my weight as the reason I couldn't give birth vaginally, which was hurtful and felt wrong. My body couldn't be the problem - I've always been athletic and strong physically, despite any pregnancy weight. It lit a fire in my heart to figure out how it all happened, with the intent of making my next birth a VBAC.
I spent almost a year researching, joining groups, attending therapy, and reading everything I could get my hands on about vaginal birth and Cesareans. All that work paid off and I've gone on to have TWO successful VBAC births, and most importantly - healed my birth trauma.

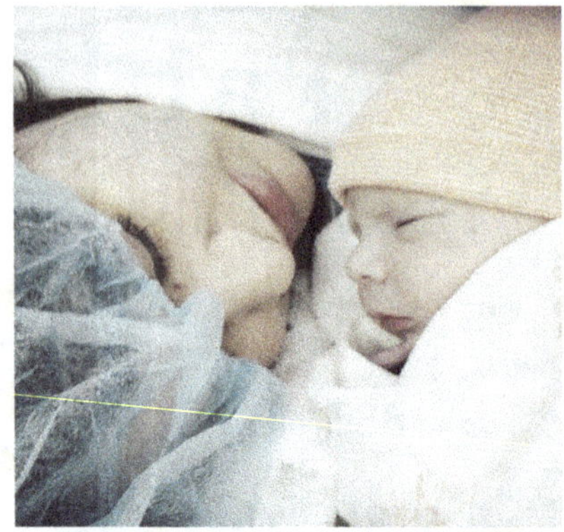

When I became a Doula I noticed a gap in the market for guides that wanted to understand the VBAC journey. The classes on the market would gladly talk about the statistics around VBAC or CBAC but were missing the key element... The birther. My hope with this course was to recenter this entire discussion around VBAC and CBAC around that astounding incredibly awesome birther. It's why we all get into this work. We witness individuals go through the ultimate feat and claim their power in so many ways.

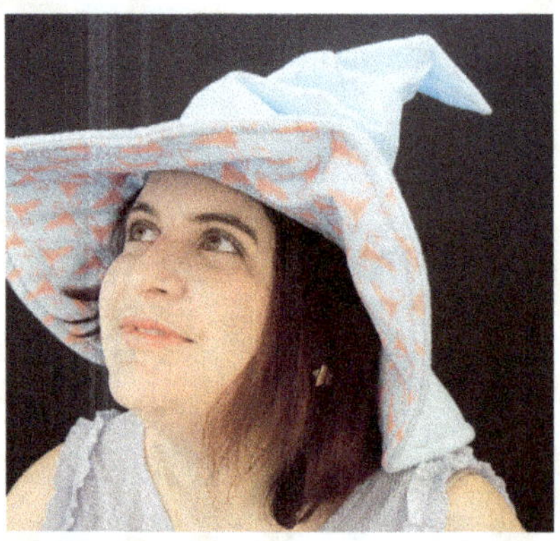

Your Birth Wizard is always excited to help with any extra assistance you need on your journey. I'm always excited to hear from participants of this course. Summon any Birth Wizard by sending an email or carrier pigeon.

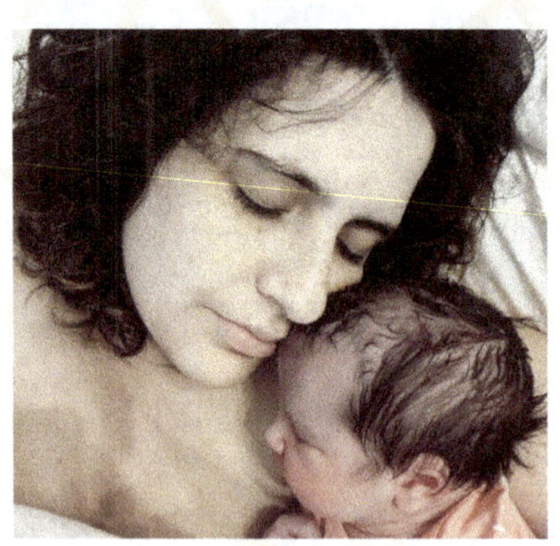

Here's to you and your future birth work and empowering others

Emmy Howard

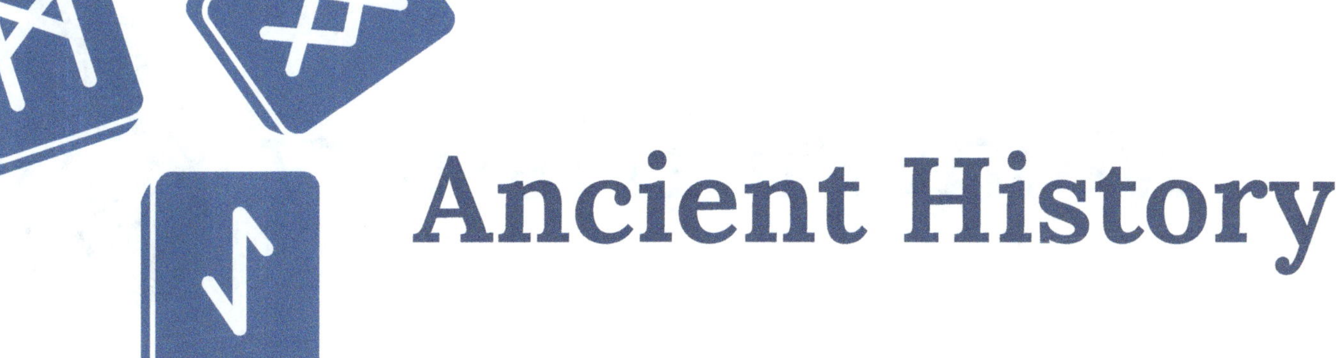

Ancient History

_____________ clan in England introduced obstetrical forceps to pull from the birth canal fetuses in _____'s

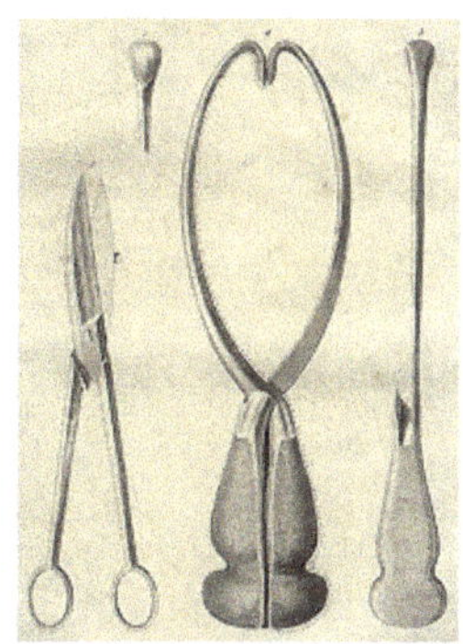

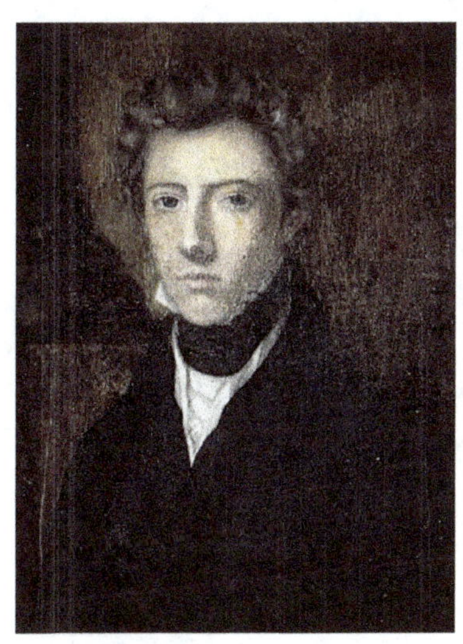

______ ______ is famous for performing first successful cesarean birth in United Kingdom

Skills he picked up from the indigenous people of _______ Kingdom

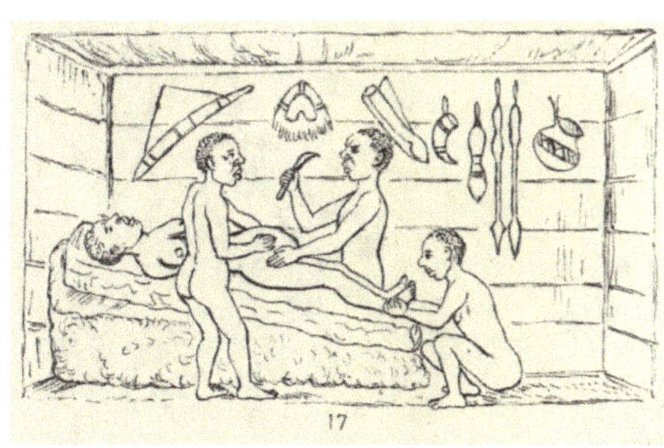

Modern History

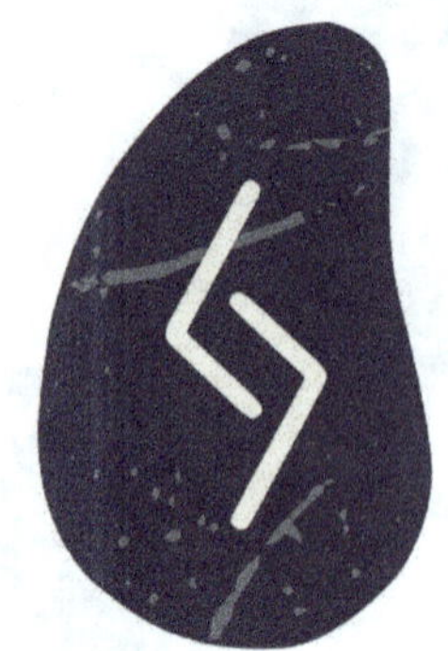

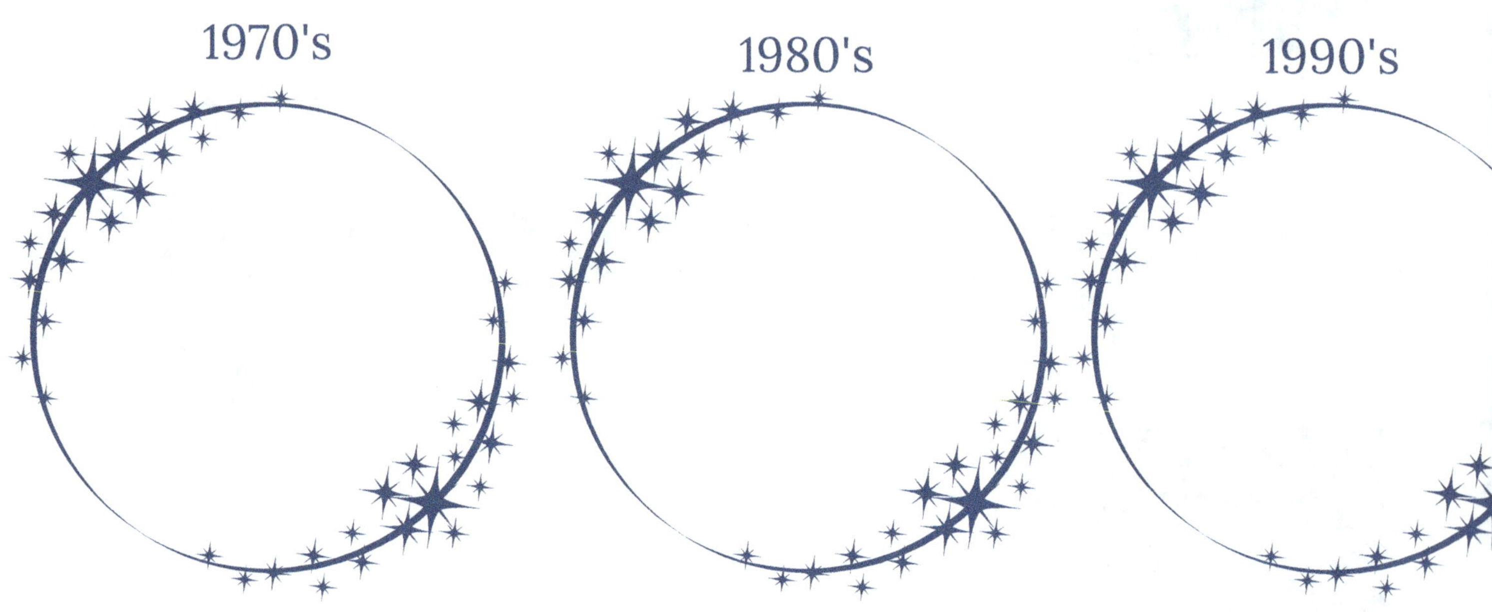

In 2018 ~__% was the national Cesarean Rate

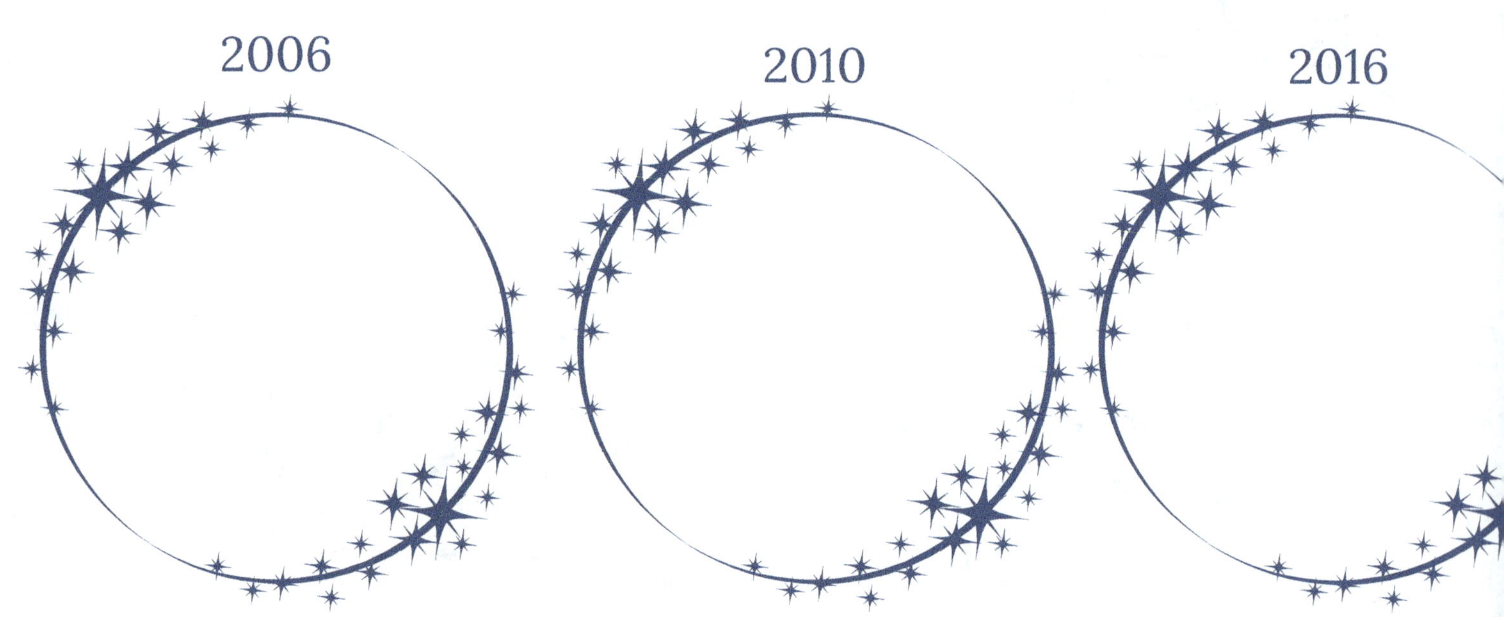

Obstacles:VBAC

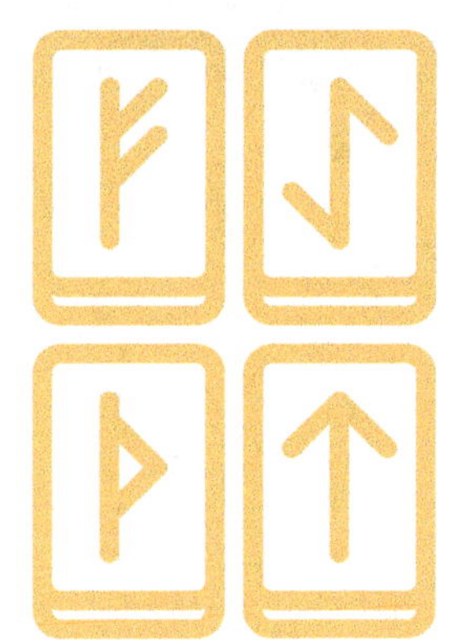

Fill in the States VBAC Laws Covered

Certified Nurse Midwives **(CNMs)**
Certified Professional Midwives **(CPMs)**

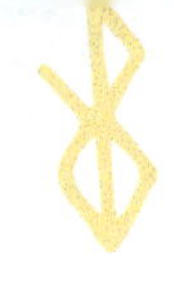

ACRONYMS

VBAC
Vaginal Birth After Cesarean

RCS
Repeat Cesarean
Individual opted for a Repeat
Cesarean without intention of VBAC

VBA#C
Vaginal Birth After # Cesarean

CBAC
Cesarean Birth After Cesarean
with the intention of a VBAC

HBAC
Home Birth After Cesarean

CBA#C
Cesarean Birth After # Cesarean
with the intention of a VBAC

Decipher the post!

Trigger warning----CBAC, bladder
injury and, baby distress.
Well I did not get the vba2c that I
was so close to getting but I am
happy my baby is here safe & sound.

____

____

How have you HBAC mamas
lovingly helped your home birth
opposed/resistant partners come
around to the idea of home birth?

____

____

HELP!
Trying to decide between a VBAC or
a RCS? How did you decide? I just
don't want to make the wrong
decision.

____

____

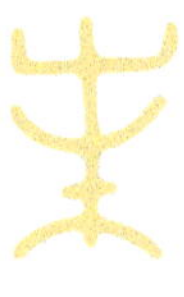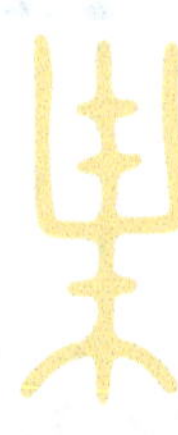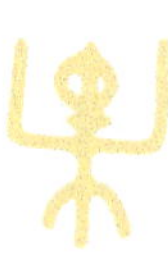

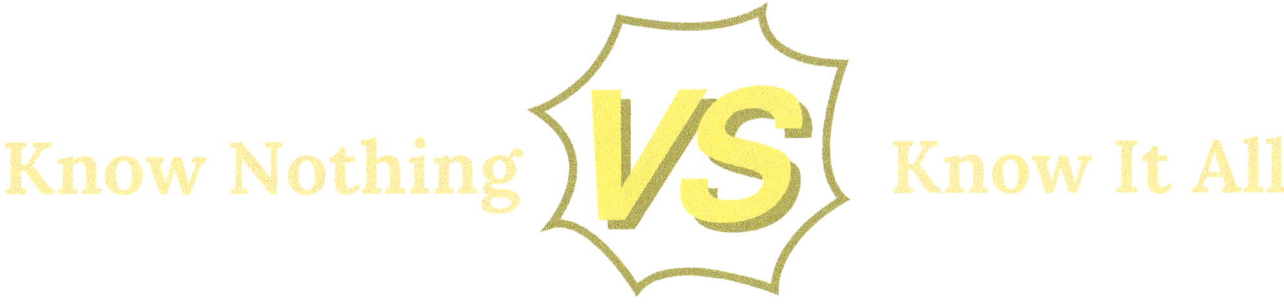

Label who is the know it all and who is the Know nothing

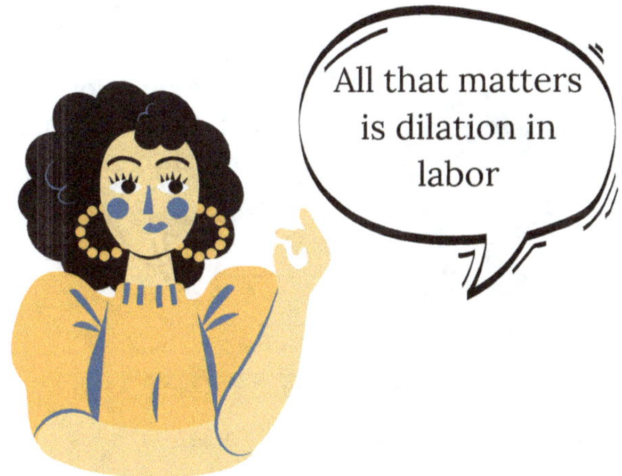

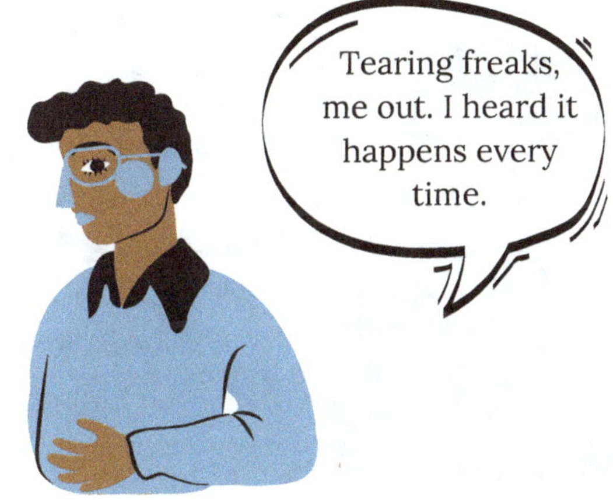

____

____

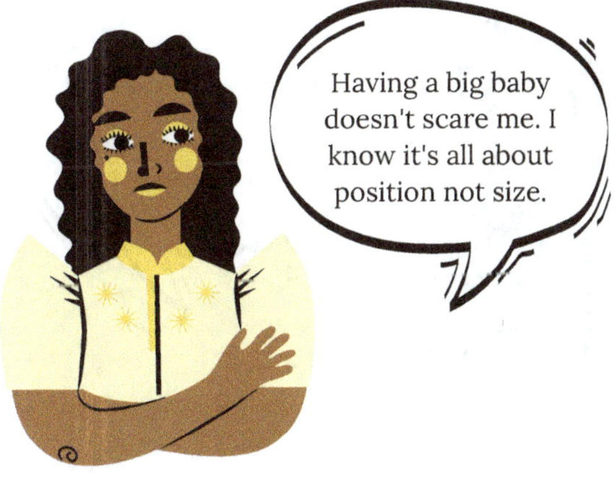

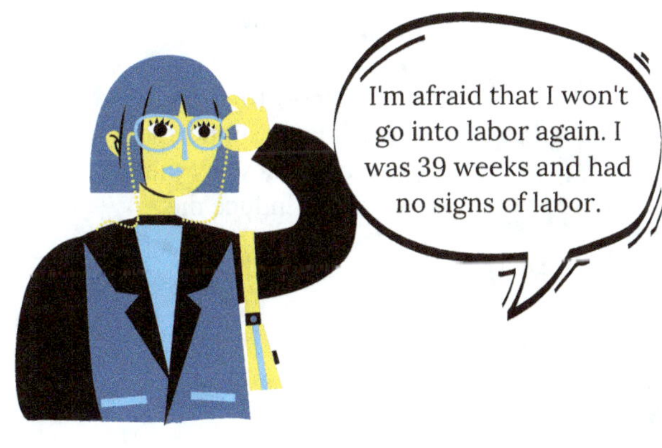

____

____

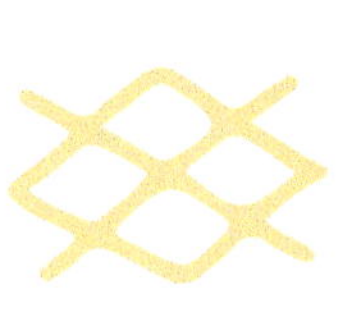

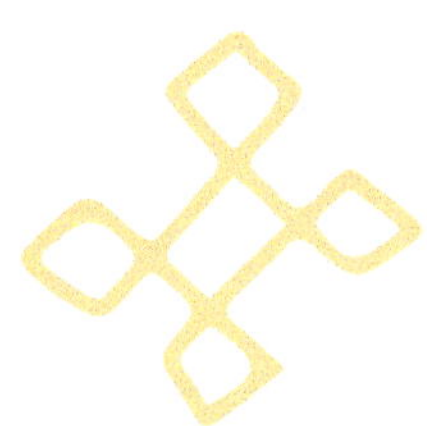

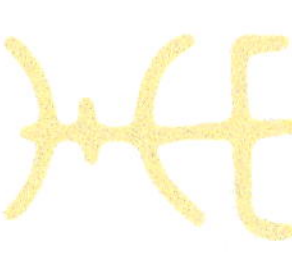

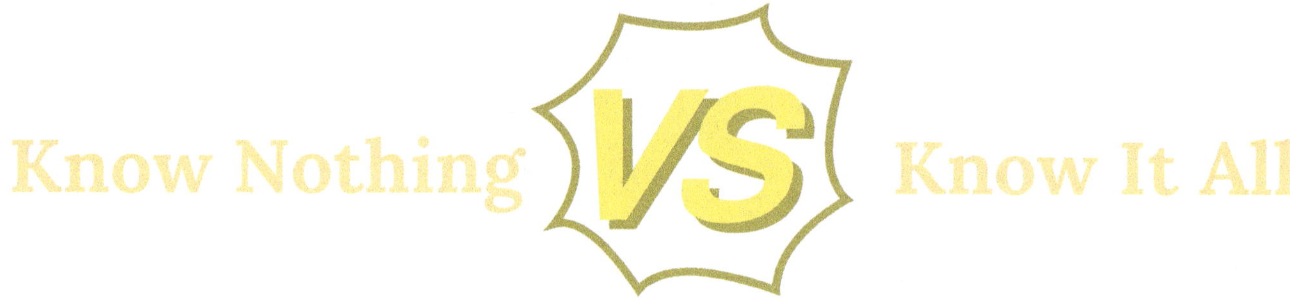

Label who is the know it all and who is the Know nothing

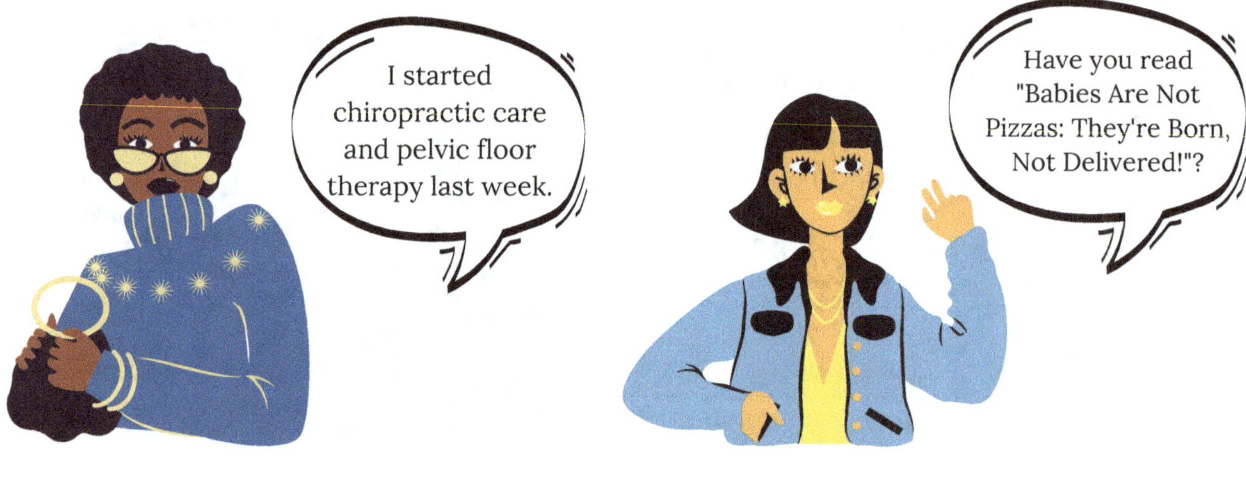

_______________________   _______________________

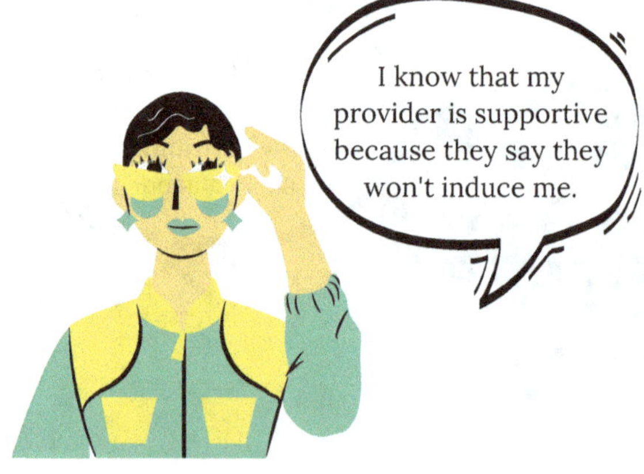

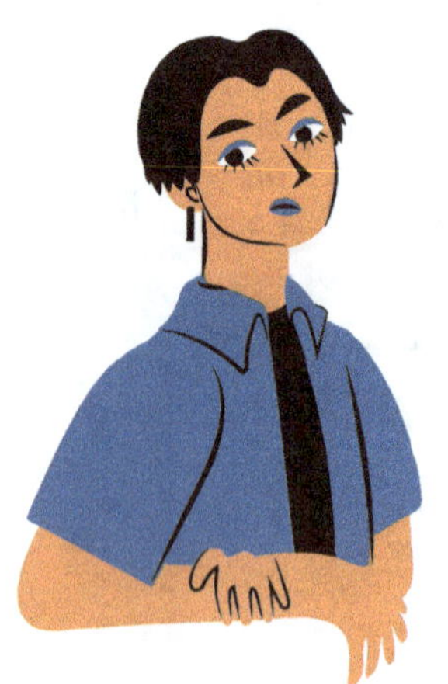

_______________________   _______________________

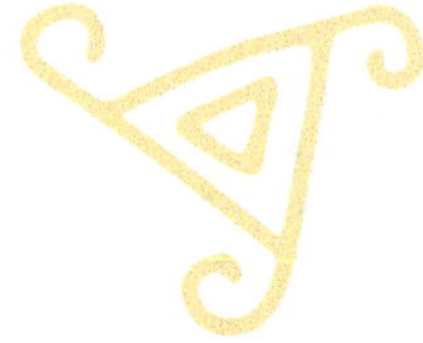
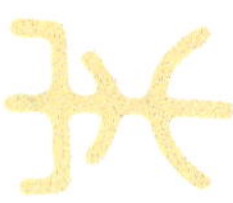

Breaking it Down

#VBAC

Yes, they are considered a VBAC still. Yes, they may still have push back from providers even with a "proven pelvis"

Vaginal Birth before they had a cesarean

This individual will have experienced a prior vaginal birth and may not need as much guidance around the mechanics of birth and more around advocacy

Cesarean after Labor

Birther went into spontaneous labor with previous birth. They may have plenty of techniques and tools to help themselves through labor but may need to process.

Cesarean without experiencing Labor

Birther never experienced labor. They may need more assistance in understanding physicological birth and may even struggle with being final on the idea of VBAC instead of RCS.

Party Members

Support from afar

____

____

____

Support up close

____

____

____

Let's Get Nerdy

VBAC Calculator

Introduced in 2007
7,600 birthers data collected

ACOG encourages the use of VBAC Calculators

What is your VBAC Calcultor Percentage?

_ _ _%

Remember that there are many factors that
go into this percentage

MFM U Network has the most updated and accurate calculator

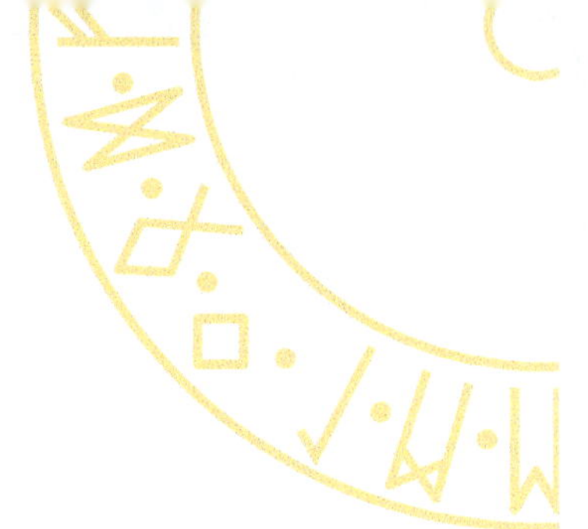
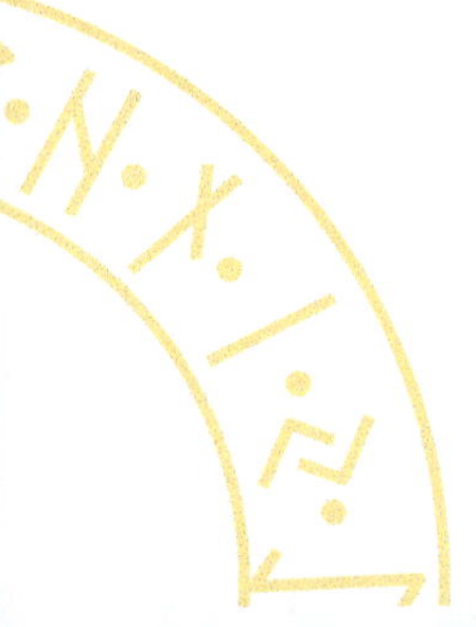

Let's Get Nerdy

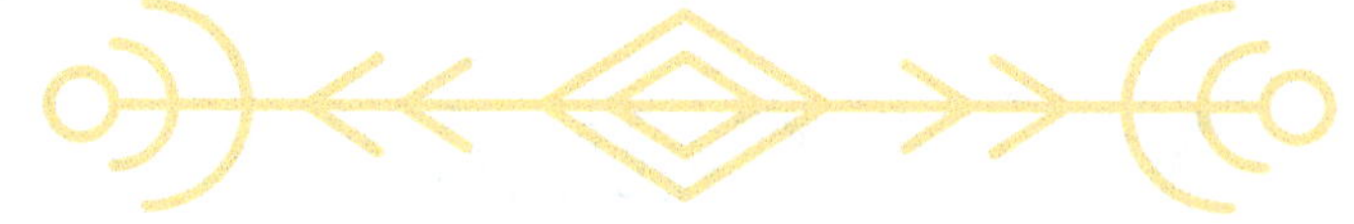

Placenta Previa

A condition in which the placenta partially or wholly blocks the neck of the uterus, thus interfering with normal delivery of a baby

Placenta Accreta

A serious pregnancy condition that occurs when the placenta grows too deeply into the uterine wall

Uterine Window

The Uterus stretches and can become thin. In order to know if there is a uterine, window, a Cesarean would need to be performed or an ultrasound may show the thinning. No evidence has not shown thus far if a U.W. is an indicator that a rupture would be more likely.

Uterine Rupture

Uterine rupture occurs when the wall of your uterus breaks open, often because of pressure caused by pregnancy. Uterine Rupture is rare and is often mistaken for dehiscence.

Uterine Dehiscence

There are 3 layers to the Uterus. If the scar opens partially, streching the scar tissue and opening the bottom layer. Uterine Dehiscence is often harmless and doesn't have any harmful effects on the baby or the mother.

Quick Guide Stats

VBAC

Successful VBAC Rate	80%
Risk of Uterine Rupture	~0.75%
Risk of Hysterectomy	0.23%
Risk of Blood Loss	1.89%

Repeat Cesarean

Risk of Hysterectomy	1.4 %
Risk of Blood Transfusion	1.53 %
Risk of Placenta Accreta	0.31 %
"Major" Complications	4.3 %
Risk of Scarring	21.6 %

Uterus Rupture

No Scar on Uterus
.007%

One Previous Cesarean
.5-.87%

Two Previous Cesarean
1.85%

Placenta Previa

No Scar on Uterus
.26%

One Previous Cesarean
.65%

Two Previous Cesarean
1.8%

Placenta Accreta

No Scar on Uterus
.24%

One Previous Cesarean
.31%

Two Previous Cesarean
.57%

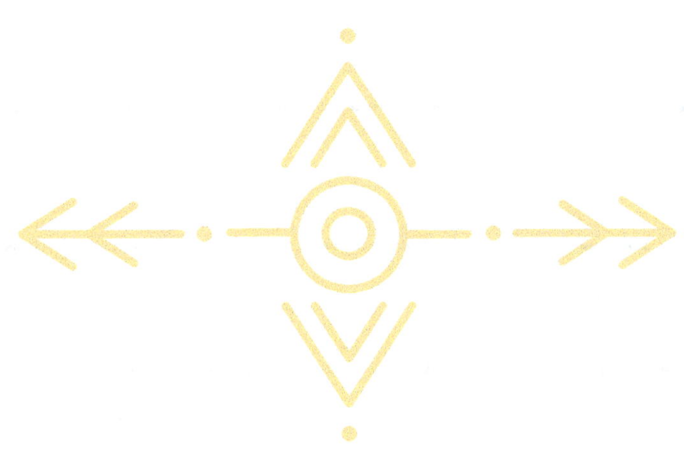

Quick Guide Stats

Uterine Rupture
~.5% or 1 in 250

Having Heart Attack
1 in 160

Dating a Millonaire
1 in 216

Having Twins
1 in 30

Risk of Cord Prolapse
1 in 300

Falling to your death
1 in 199

Audited by the IRS
1 in 160

Come up with 4 examples of situations

____

____

____

____

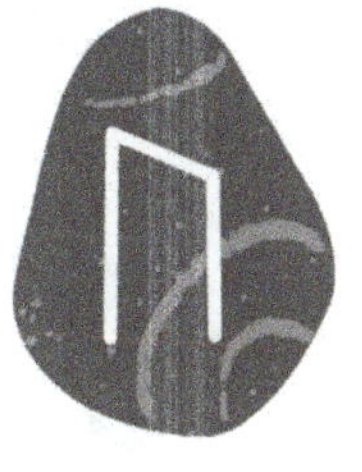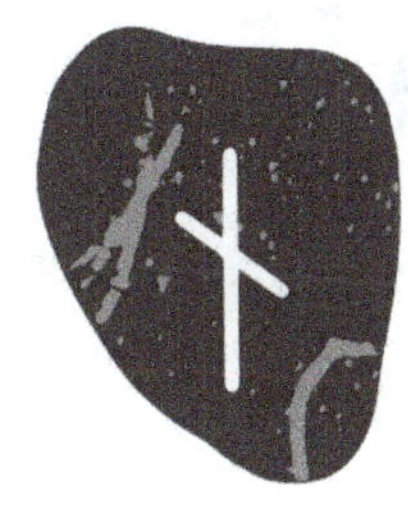

Scars

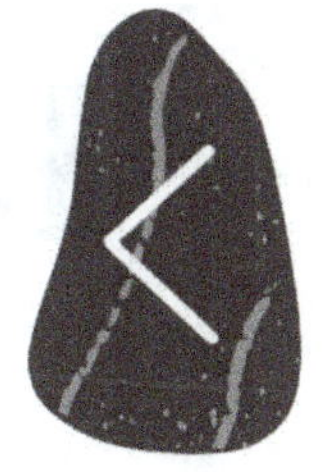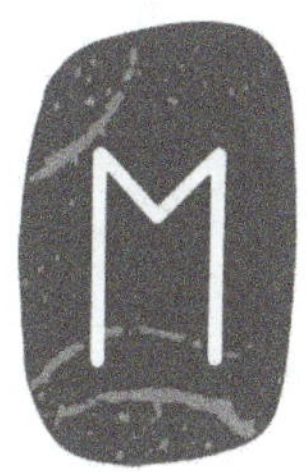

C-section Incision Types

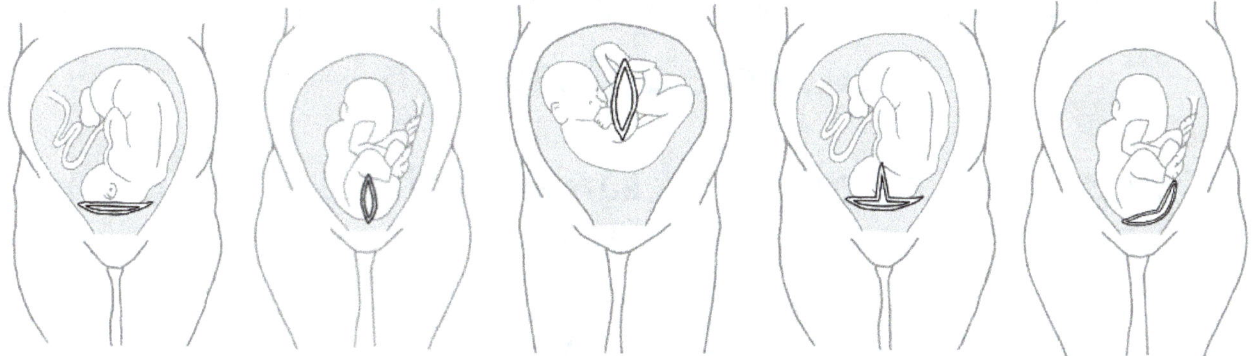

Low Vertical

____

Low Transverse

____

Classical

____

Inverted T and J

____

Unknown Incision Types

____

Race & VBAC

Birthers of Color are significantly more likely to have a Cesarean

Twice of as likely to have Cesarean births than white, non hispanic birthers

Die of Cesarean Birth Complications

Black, American Indian, and Alaska Native (AI/AN) birthers are two to three times more likely to die from pregnancy-related causes than white birthers

Birthers of Color are significantly less likely to have a successful VBAC

Analysis of over 100,000 births, this study shows that white, non-hispanic birthers are almost 10% more likely to have a successful VBAC than black, non-Hispanic

Provider

MFM

A maternal-fetal medicine specialist is a doctor who helps take care of women having complicated or high-risk pregnancies

OBGYN

A Obstetrician-gynecologist is a healthcare professional that specializes in female reproductive health

CNM

A nurse-midwife is a licensed healthcare professional who specializes in women's reproductive health and childbirth

CPM

Certified Professional Midwife (CPM) is a knowledgeable, skilled and professional independent midwifery practitioner who has met the standards for certification set by the North American Registry of Midwives (NARM) and is qualified to provide the Midwives Model of Care

Unlicensed Midwife

Traditional midwife who is trained informally but gained education and knowledge of all things birth through apprenticeship or self-study.

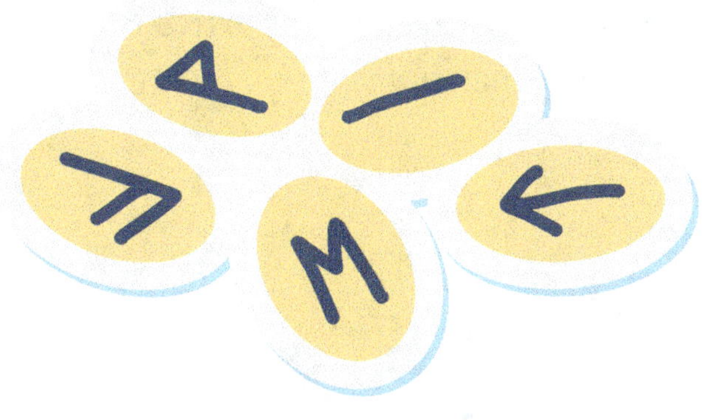

Put it to the test

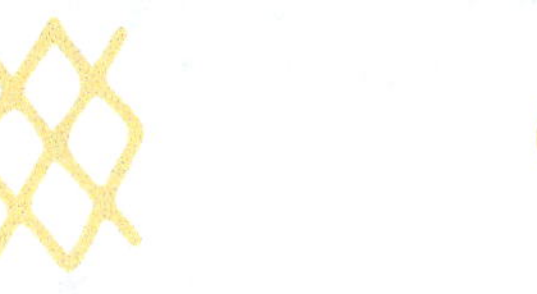
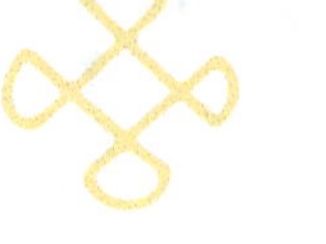
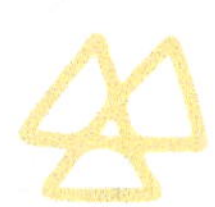
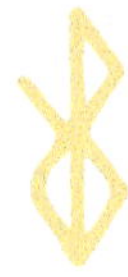

Safe

- [ ] No arbitrary restrictions on length of gestation
- [ ] Induction or augmentation are options if medically necessary or advisable
- [ ] No weight guesstimates used to discourage you from VBAC
- [ ] As long as Birther and baby are doing well, labor does not have time limits
- [ ] Encourages laboring outside of the hospital longer to avoid unnecessary interventions
- [ ] Low cesarean and high VBAC rates
- [ ] Supports VBAmC
- [ ] Can guarantee that they, or an equally supportive provider will be the one to attend your birth

Unsafe

- [ ] Must go into labor by Due date
- [ ] Won't induce or augment under any circumstance
- [ ] Baby must be under X lbs
- [ ] Must progress X cm/hr
- [ ] Must come to the hospital in early labor
- [ ] Epidural placed "just in case"
- [ ] Internal fetal monitoring and/or intrauterine pressure catheter required
- [ ] Must have double layer sutures
- [ ] Uses a VBAC calculator
- [ ] Shares a practice with other unsupportive providers that don't share their view and may not "let you"

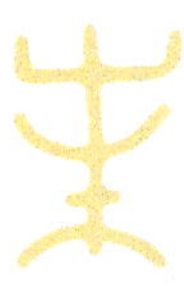
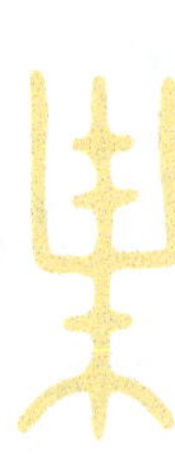
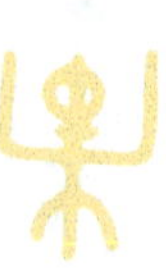

Provider List

Take a moment to chat with the class and get some providers on your list

Bag of Holding

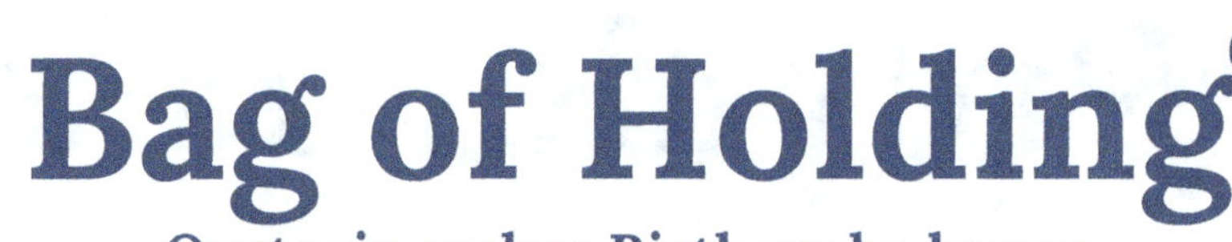

Oxytocin makes Birthers be happy
Happy Birthers bring babies...
they just do
What are your favorite ways to get oxytocin going?

No Go

Cyotec/Cervidil

Not Safe for use in VBAC.
Study done with 512 birthers attempting VBAC, 5.6% of women receiving Misoprostol had symptomatic uterine rupture compared to .2% of birthers having a Trail of Labor without Misoprostol.

Evening Primrose Oil

Not recommended for VBAC without Medical oversight
Two studies available and both didn't show progression of labor and did get linked to bleeding issues and complications during Cesareans.

Castor Oil

Not recommended for VBAC without Medical oversight
There has only been one study done on induction and castor oil. In that study, one birther had a U.R. when attempting her VBAC.

Tool Bag

Foley Blub

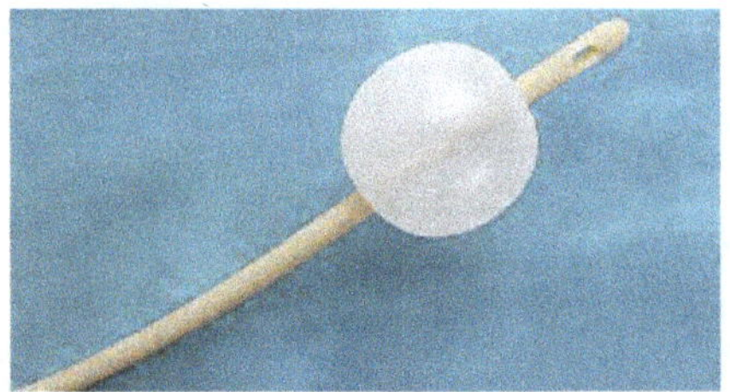

A small catheter that is inserted into the cervix. Will fall out 5 cm. May take time and can be paired with Pitocin.

Cook's Catheter

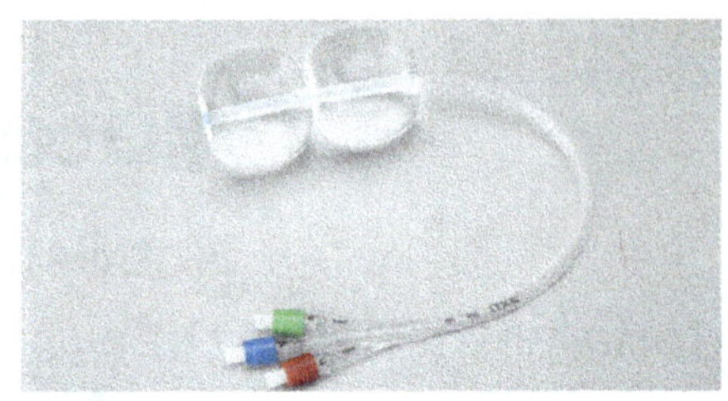

Used for mechanical dilation of the cervical canal prior to labor induction at term when the cervix is unfavorable for induction

Artificial Rupture Waters

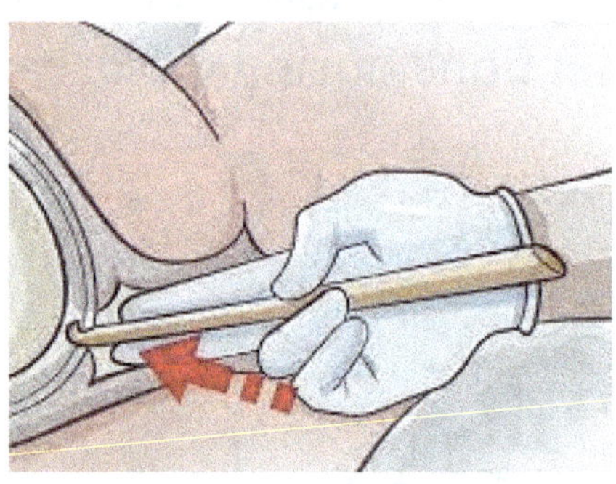

Provider inserts a long needle instrument to puncture amniotic sac. This can quicken the labor process but also removes extra cushion for baby.

Membrane Sweep

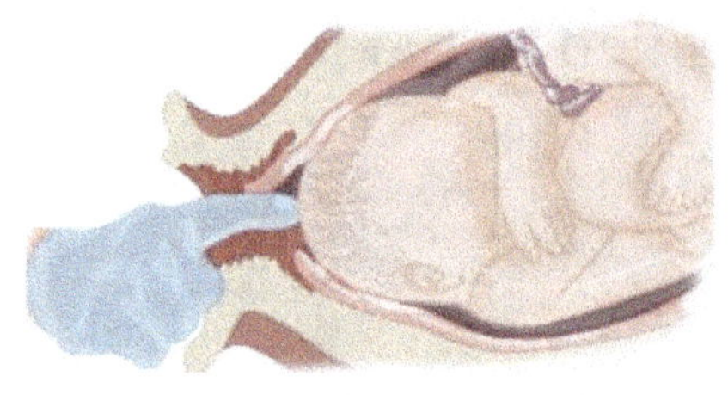

Provider inserts fingers into cervix and separates the amniotic sac from your uterine wall.

Pitocin

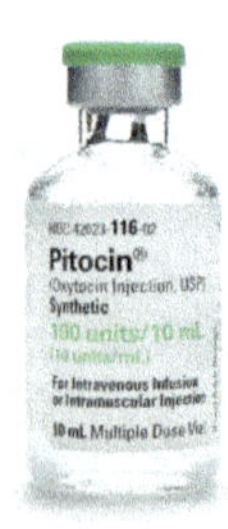

Synthetic version of Oxytocin and is administered via IV. Starts on lowest dose for VBAC 1ml and slowly upped until regular contractions. Continuous Monitoring required for VBAC.

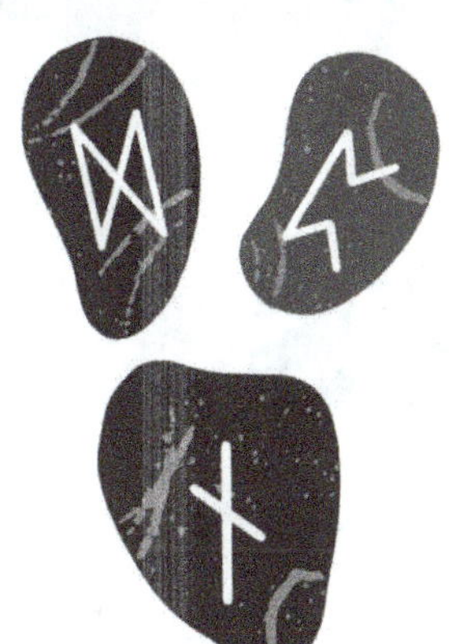

Induction

Match the Intervention

BONUS: Circle the interventions that should never be used if you are going for a VBAC

Pitocin

Anesthetic placed in spine; reduces or sometimes eliminates the ability to move on your lower half. Can cause blood pressure issues; can stall labor-especially if given too soon.

AROM/Amniotomy

An amnihook is used to break the waters within the uterus. Studies show this does not reduce the time spent in labor.

Epidural

Synthetic version of oxytocin; disrupts the body's natural wave of hormones-BUT-can be responsibly when needed

Continuous Fetal Monitoring

Infused the uterus with sterile saline to increase the water around the baby improving the cushion baby is in the womb. Can improve cord compression scenarios.

Amnioinfusion

Care provider tells Birther to start pushing based on dilation vs waiting for the Birther to feel "Pushy". Can lead to long pushing and failure to descends.

Sweeping Membranes

A surgical cut to the perineum and the muscle beneath it during the pushing stage. Can be done necessarily but is often done to reduce pushing time. Can cause scarring and other nerve damage.

Directed Pushing

Lower your chances of needing a formal induction if your pregnancy goes on too long and you and your care provider decide that you want a formal induction. This can help prevent needing medications for an induction. 9% of mothers will have their water break at the same time.

Episiotomy

Your baby's heartbeat is checked all the time. Elastic belts hold two flat devices (called sensors) on your belly. One sensor records the baby's heart rate. The other shows how long your contractions last.

Tips & Tricks

TO GETTING HIRED

STORYTELLING

Have them tell their story first

ASSESS

Do you have a
Know it all or Know Nothing

INVESTIGATE

Often context is needed to be provided to their
birth story

CONSTRUCT AUTHORITY

Your answers around their birth story and your
knowledge

WEALTH OF KNOWLEDGE

Provide resources to help them along the
journey but keep it vague

YOUR OWN FLAIR

Sell you because YOU are FANTASTIC

Unpacking Safely

Circle the techniques for unpacking safely

Reassuring client that nothing will happen because you are their doula

Be aware of your own trauma/triggers

The client needs to lead

Pushing an issue client wants to avoid

Grounding/Fear Release techniques

You taking lead of conversation

All emotions are valid

Active Listening

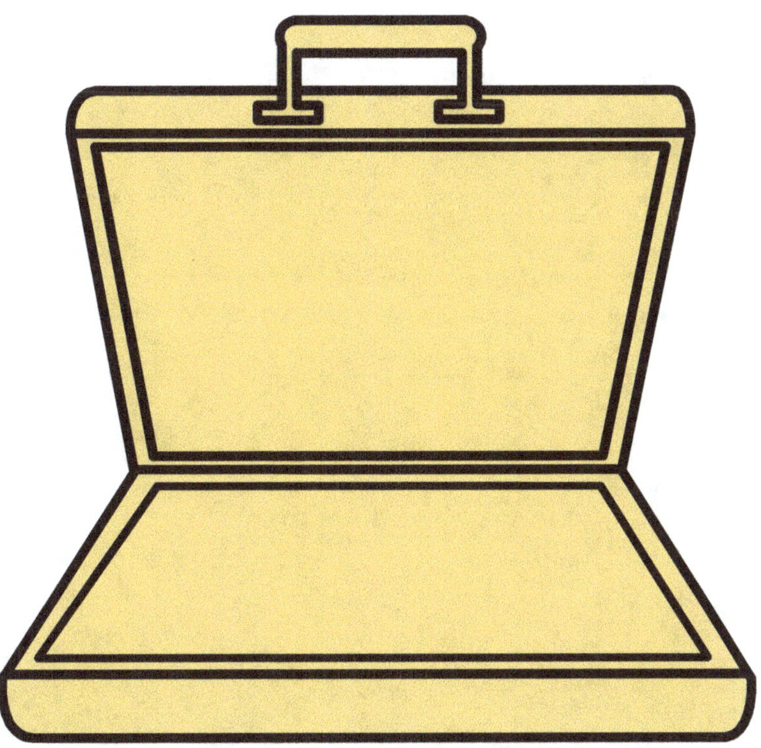

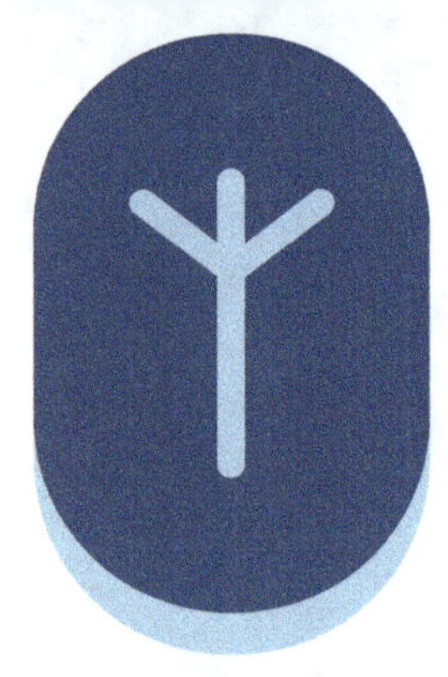 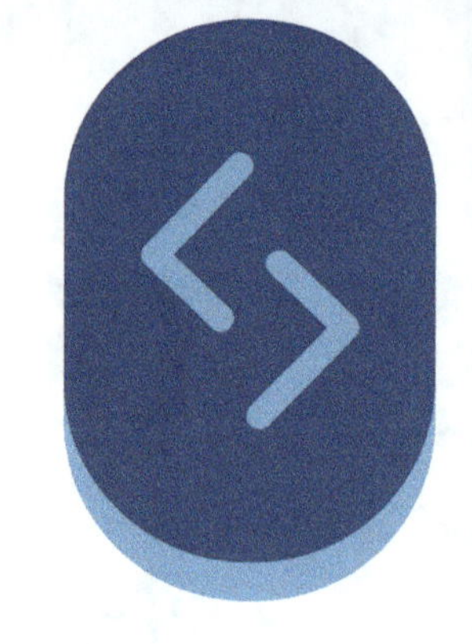

SETTING GOALS

Listen to instructor ideal birth
What goals can you pull from the
description?

Advocating

B _______________

R _______________

A _______________

I _______________

N _______________

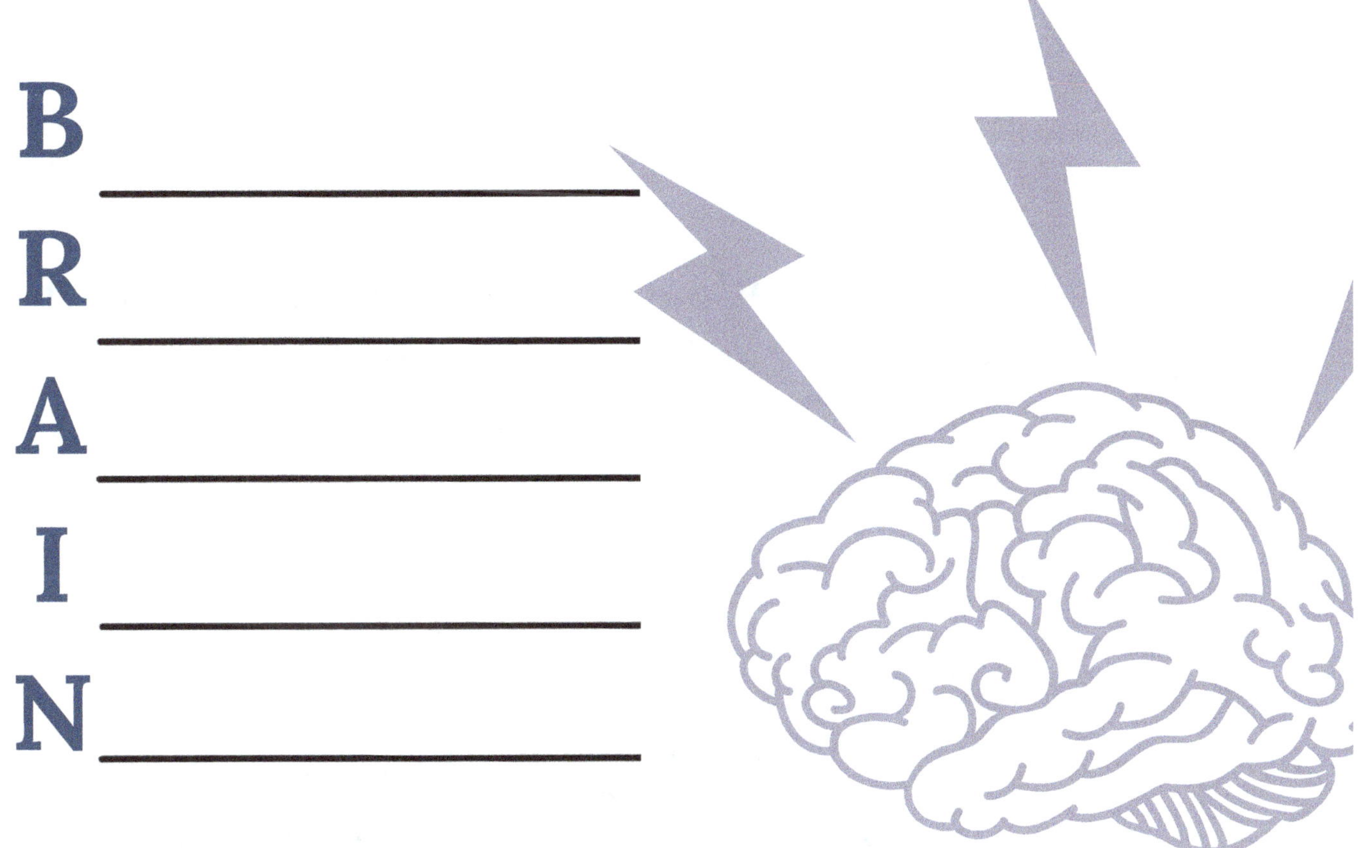

Boundary Riffing

Write down your favorites

____

____

____

____

Failure Language

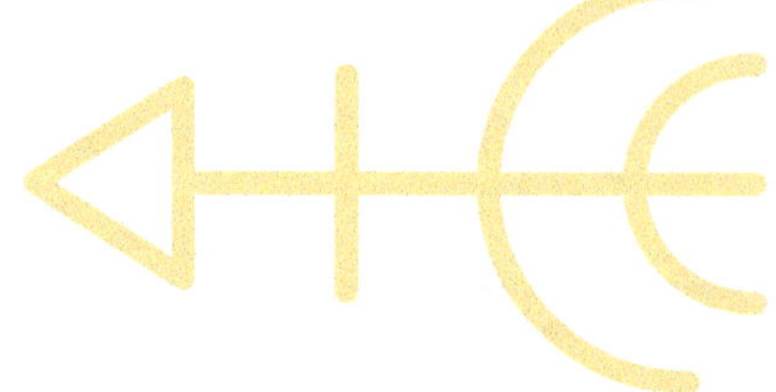

No matter what people tell you, words and ideas
can change the world.
Robin Williams

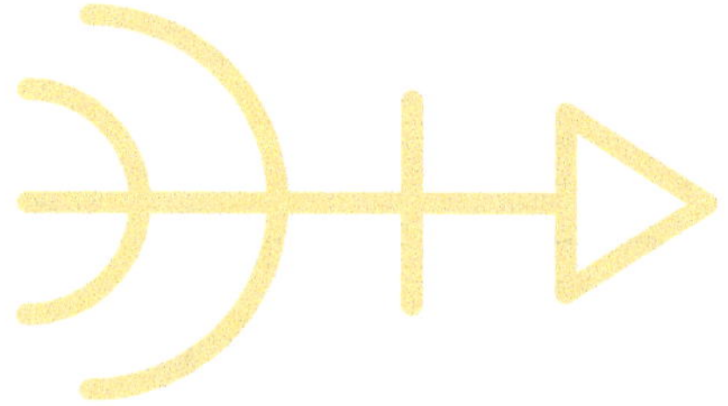

What we say matters...
During the unpacking you might hear
failure language
"My body failed."
It might not be so direct
"If had waited then this wouldn't happen"
Remember, not always is it the provider
using the language
but it might be **self inflicted**

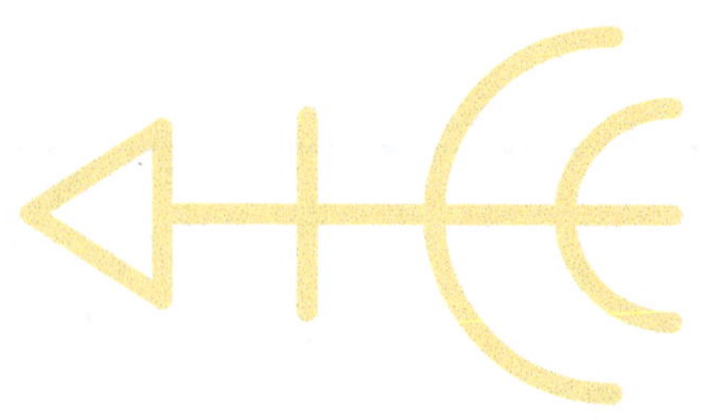

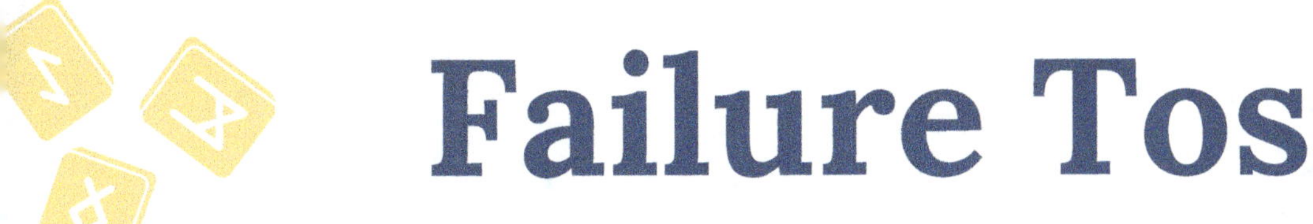

Failure Toss

Define Failure

____

____

Failure   Wisdom

Cesarean Talk

CESAREAN BIRTH IS BIRTH

They aren't to be feared. You have choices around how baby comes into this world

HEADSPACE IS KEY

Going into this birth with confident and tools of advocation will guarantee a different headspace

DISCUSS CHOICES

This prenatal allows you to go over possible choices. Then encourage talk with provider at 37 week appointment and onward

AVOID TRAUMA

You are having this discussion to avoid trauma. The Cesarean will be happening because of their choice and not to them.

LEAD WITH CONFIDENCE

Provide resources to help them along the journey.

YOU ARE DOING YOUR JOB

You are doing the kindest thing by having this discussion

BABY

VAGINAL SEEDING
A swab to capture the flora to give to baby to help their gut

SKIN TO SKIN
Guaranteed to satisfy you!

DELAYED CORD CLAMPING
Allows for all the goodness from placenta to pass to baby by around 3 minutes after birth

BIRTHER

CLEAR DRAPE
A scrumptious classic, available at most hospitals but a good substitute is having baby peep over drape.

ESSENTIAL OILS & MUSIC
Double comfort measures for birther that can keep space more tranquil

NODES PLACED ON BACK
This allows for ease of movement and breastfeeding

PHOTOGRAPHY
Memories and honoring the moment with snapshots

SLIENCE
Not hearing the OR staff talk about their kid's soccer practice or upcoming vacation can keep the mood on point

SUPPORT

DOULA IN OR
The perfect sweetness to add to any OI

PARTNER STAYING WITH BABY
Our best-seller! This is an easy request that can fulfilled just about everytime.

BE SURE TO TALK

PROVIDER ABOUT THEIR SECRET MEN

Fear Release

Brains are great story tellers and the body is it hype man. We as doulas are here to teach birthers when to engage with the story, quiet the hype man and bring peace to the swirly thoughts.

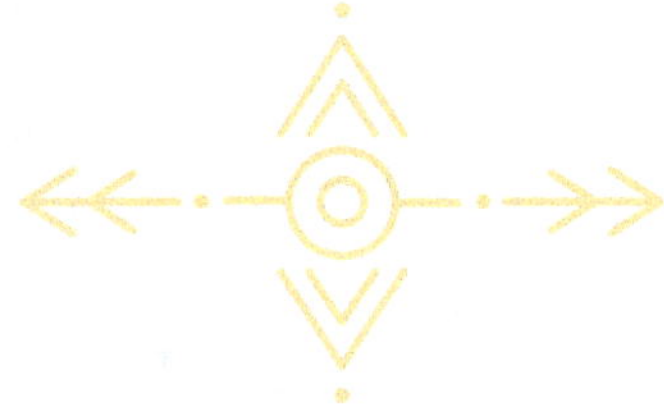

There is so much information that can seem contradictory when nunation isn't introduced

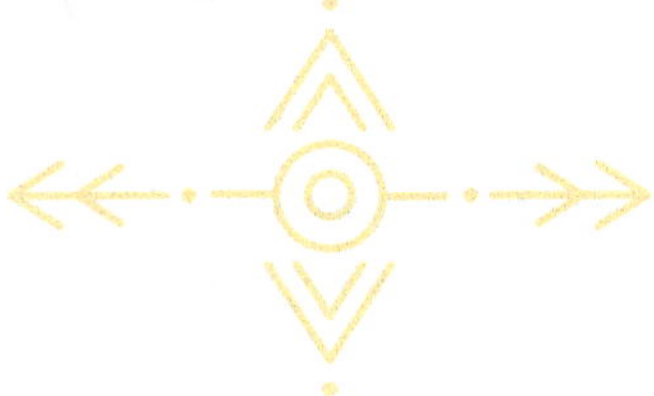

Logic + Heart + Kinect

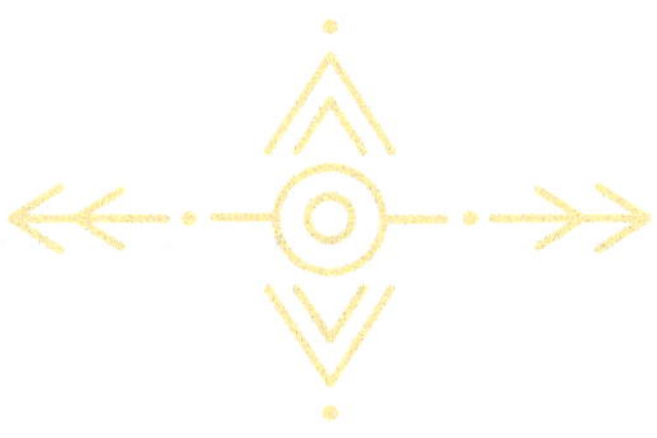

Fear Release

Fear Bubbles

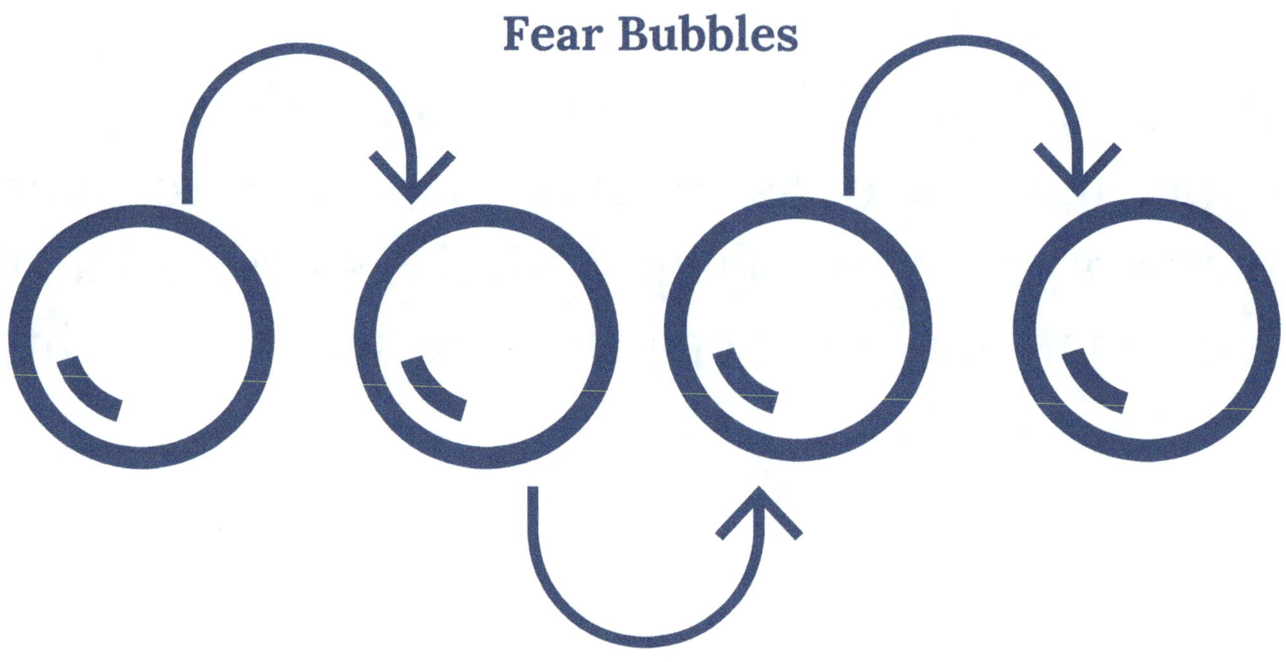

Breath Work

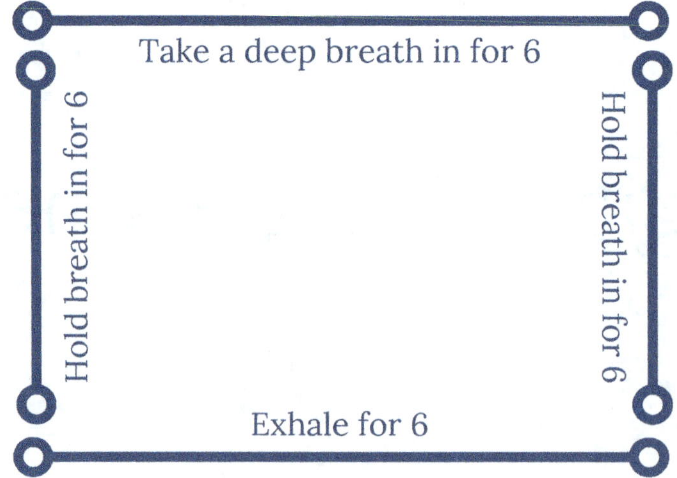

Mental Games

Catastrophe Game

____
____
____
____
____
____
____
____

Nothing Changes

____
____
____
____
____
____
____
____

It's not a "real" birth

____
____
____
____
____

Game of your own

____
____
____
____
____

Birth Trauma

Stats say ___ birthing people will have a traumatic birth

Who is at risk?

___________ complications
Birthing Interventions
Babies needing _________ care
People with significant injuries
People with existing _______ problems
People with previous trauma and abuse People from marginalized backgrounds
NO ONE IS IMMUNE!!

___ of people try a treatment approach and it doesn't work

Write 4 resources you can use in case of emergency

____

____

____

____

Anticipation

There is no terror in the bang, only in the
anticipation of it
- **Alfred Hitchcock**

Patience is not the ability to wait, but the ability to keep a good
attitude while waiting

This is the hardest part

Be creative about how to get them distracted

Utilized active listening

Fear release might have to be revisited a couple times

Write 4 suggestions you can use to encourage distraction

____

____

____

____

____

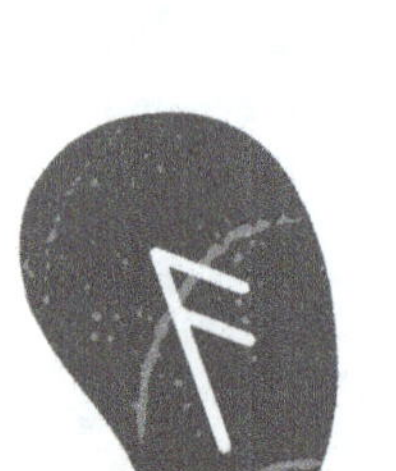

Prodromal Labor

Prodrome is a medical term for early signs or symptoms of an illness or health problem that appear before the major signs or symptoms start

What are the symptoms of prodromal labor?

____

____

____

____

How can you use it to guide your client?

____

____

____

____

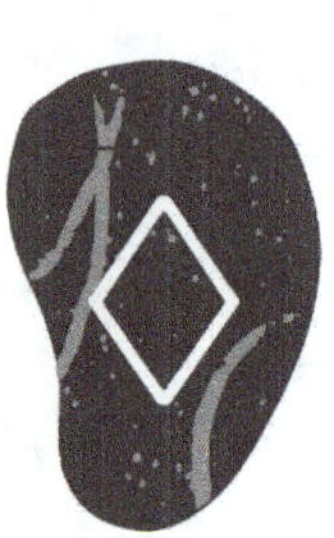

"I'm over this"

What are some key lines you can pick up from the script that could help you flip the mindset?

Support

Wants you there

This is those moments where VBACs can feel like first time birthers

Signs of impending labor might be seen as sound the alarms

Find 4 ways for you to check in and assess client

____

____

____

____

OR

Is very quiet

This is those moments where VBACs can feel like old pros

Signs of Impeding labor will be ignored and put themselves in denial

Find 4 ways for you to check in and assess client

____

____

____

____

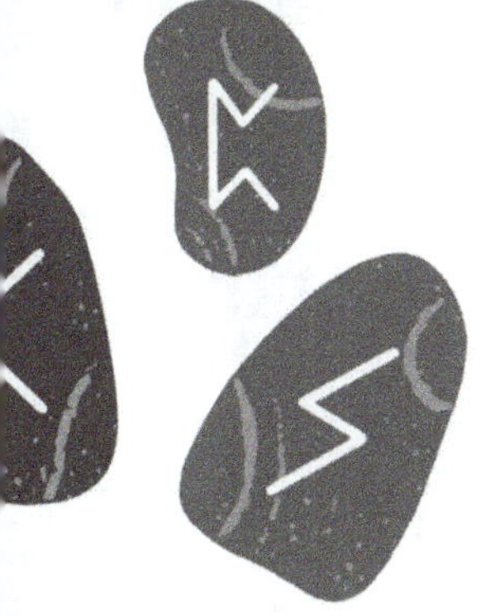

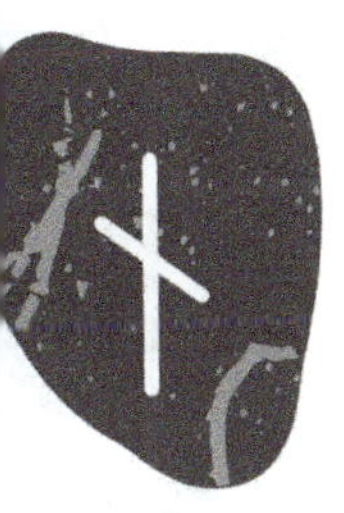

PUSHING

sur·re·al
/səˈrēəl/
adjective
1. having the qualities of surrealism; bizarre.
2.   "a surreal mix of fact and fantasy"

Guidance for pushing might be more intense
Client will need that bringing into self
Surreal is a word said most often
**Expect for you to have an emotional
response**

**Name 4 tools to help client
with connecting body and mind during pushing**

____

____

____

____

Focus

What control do they have

What goals have they hit

How Joyous this moment is

Highs & Lows

Supporting Birthers in goal of a redemptive or
healing birth has a lot of weight put on the outcome
and your service.
There is the inspiring and magical births that are
total highs
There is also the heartbreaking and tragic births
that bring you crashing down
Sometimes they loop around to bring unexpecting
twists
You being there made a difference
Prepare yourself for the twists and turns

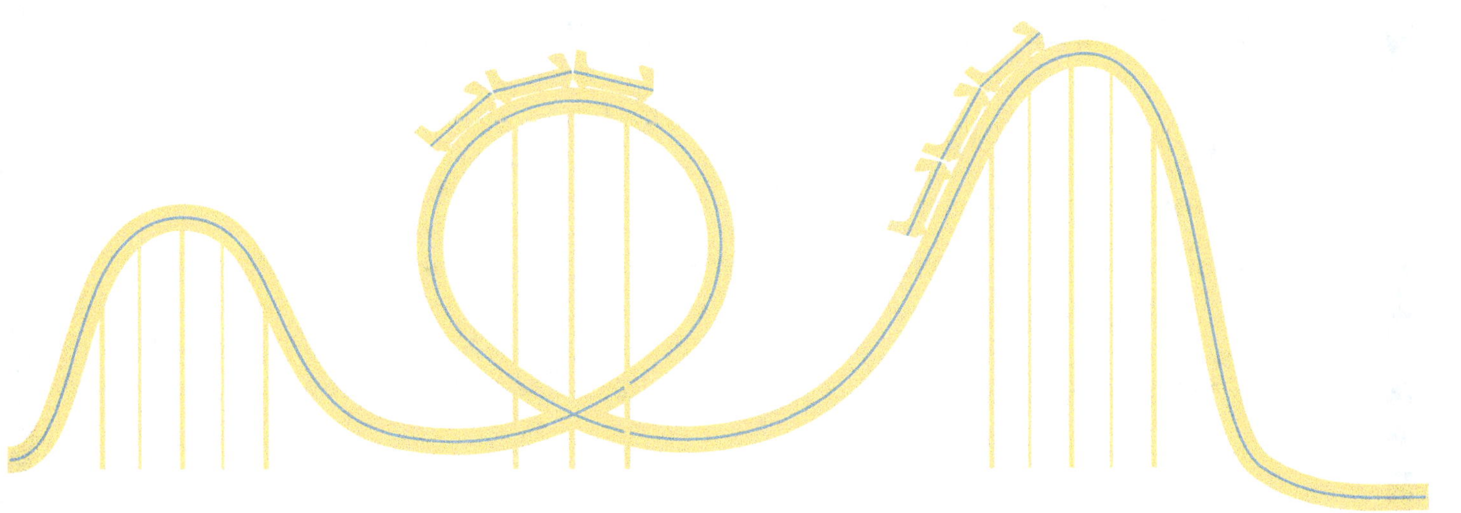

Self-Care Checklist

because you deserve it

Before

- Sleep
- Meditation
- Therapy
- Creative Expressive
- Time with peers
- Kinect output

During

- Eat
- Use the bathroom
- Rest when birther rests
- Stretch
- Leave when tired

Directly after

- Play Tetris
- Emergency Playlist for laughs
- Call peer to process
- Sing/Yell
- Essential Oil

After

- Sleep
- Eat
- Creative Expressive
- Kinect Output
- Treat yourself

Educating Community

Be the resource
Be the ADVOCATE
BE THE GUIDE

Name 4 ways you can educate your community about VBAC or CBAC

____

____

____

____

Presenting of your Certificate of Birth Wisdom

DOODLES & NOTES

DOODLES & NOTES

DOODLES & NOTES

DOODLES & NOTES

LET'S DRAW

Draw a picture of your birth. Put everything from smells, sounds, lighting, colors, feelings.. be abstract

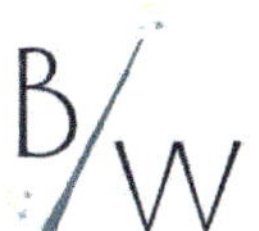

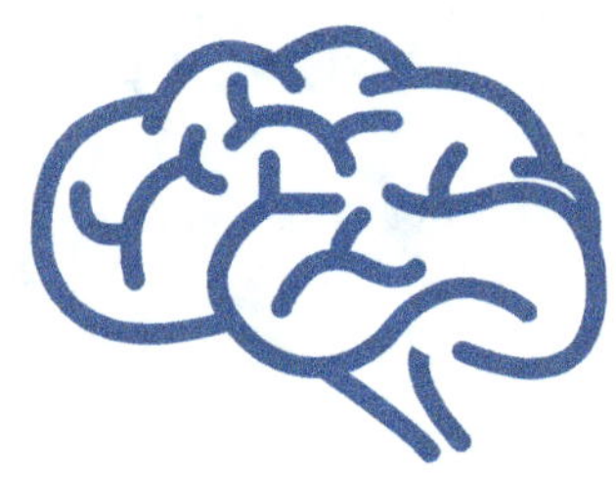

FIRST
THING
THAT
COMES
TO MIND

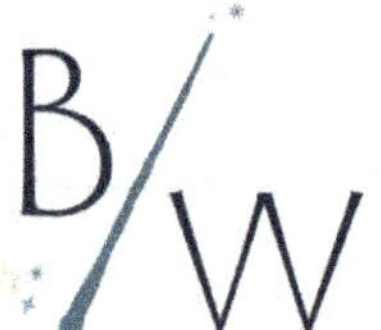

Cesarean Birth

Discuss with your Birth Wizard

Your Previous Cesarean Birth

One Thing I need to know

One Thing I want to know

www.ingramcontent.com/pod-product-compliance
Lightning Source LLC
Chambersburg PA
CBHW081601270726
48657CB00029B/3447